CBD: 101 Things You Need To Know About CBD Oil

Frank Coles

Table of Contents

Introduction

Congratulations on downloading *"CBD: 101 Things You Need to Know About CBD Oil!"*

This book was designed to shed as much light on CBD Oil as possible. From supporting you in understanding what the supplement is and where it comes from to discovering why it is used and what side effects you may face when using it, this guide contains everything. It truly is the most comprehensive guide on the market to support you in understanding CBD Oil and how it can positively benefit you or your loved ones who are considering using it.

CBD Oil has been recognized and studied since it was discovered more than half a century ago. In that time, researchers have discovered fascinating information about this supplement and what it can do for our health. If you are ready to learn all about the supplement that everyone is talking about, this book is exactly the right place to be. You are going to learn all that there is to know.

One important thing when it comes to our health

is recognizing that being well-informed is necessary. With supplements such as CBD Oil, which is still illegal in many places, the information shared online and in the media can be highly controversial. Many are still morally against it based on the nature of its origin, whereas, other more liberal people are extremely excited by it and the many things it can do for us and our health.

Educating yourself and making sure that you are well-informed about the truth can support you in making a choice that works for *your* health. Remember, what goes into your body needs to be right for *you*. So, stay informed and make the best choice for yourself.

Now, if you are ready to get informed, get ready to be impressed! You will not find anything as comprehensive as this online, all in one place. This is the perfect book to support beginners in educating themselves on the values of this supplement and how it works. If you are ready to learn more, begin! And of course, enjoy!

Chapter 1: What is CBD Oil?

These are the essential facts you need to know about what CBD Oil is and where it comes from. These facts will help you understand the history of CBD Oil, what part of the plant it is extracted from, and how this contributes to the Oil working in your body.

What is CBD Oil?

1st thing you need know...

CBD is one of at least 113 unique cannabinoid chemical compounds found in Cannabis and Hemp Plants. This list is not believed to be exhausted as scientists are regularly discovering new cannabinoid chemical compounds on regular basis. Many of these compounds are either irrelevant or are still being researched so that they can be applied in modern and alternative medicine.

2nd thing you need know...

Although CBD is found in Cannabis plants, THC is the most common and abundantly found cannabinoid present in Cannabis. In reverse, THC is found only in trace amounts in Hemp plants whereas CBD is the dominant, naturally occurring component.

3rd thing you need know...

Cannabidiol is known to account for up to 40% of the extracts derived from the Hemp plant. Other extracts include Hemp Oil and Hemp Seed Oil, each of which is used for different purposes.

Hemp Seed Oil is well known for having a healthy fatty acid profile which promotes healing. This means that Hemp Seed Oil is often used for treating inflammation and is good for various skin conditions such as eczema. Whereas, Hemp Oil is still typically used for CBD Oil.

4th thing you need know...

Despite being a relative of THC, the compound in marijuana that gets you high, CBD is not an addictive compound.

Unlike THC, CBD interacts naturally with our internal systems without being psychotropic, meaning it doesn't get you high. This important biochemical feature of CBD makes it a safer treatment option than medical Marijuana.

5th thing you need know...

CBD is classified as a "food supplement" in many countries. This means that when taking it, you are not actually ingesting a form of what is considered to be a drug, but rather, you are taking a natural supplement.

CBD has many great medical benefits, which I will discuss in "*Chapter 2: Why Should I Use CBD Oil?.*"

6th thing you need know...

In recent years CBD has gained in popularity due to its many benefits such as relief from chronic pain and ailments such as seizure disorders.

7th thing you need know...

Despite not being able to get you high, CBD Oil will cause significant changes in your body. These changes are caused by the cannabinoids attaching themselves to your endocannabinoid system, allowing them to regulate functions which support relief from pain and other difficult or debilitating symptoms.

8th thing you need know...

Hemp is the least processed form of a Cannabis plant. It also happens to be the plant that contains the highest volume of CBD that can be extracted and used for medical benefits such as anxiety, epilepsy, nausea and cancer.

9th thing you need know...

Despite both coming from the Cannabis Sativa plant, Hemp and Marijuana are two very different things. They both have different genetics based on being different strains of the same plant. Also, they are cultivated for different uses.

Historically, and due to historical laws, Hemp was a legal crop that could be grown for the creation of fibers such as cloth and paper. Marijuana, however, has been outlawed in most countries for quite some time and is not typically used for anything beyond its psychoactive effects.

10th thing you need know...

Marijuana farmers have spent a long time selectively breeding Marijuana strains to increase THC levels in their plants. Hemp farmers, on the other hand, have barely altered the plant at all. This means that these plants are still incredibly high in CBD Oil, hence why most CBD Oil comes from hemp farmers.

11th thing you need know...

CBD Oil is present in Hemp Oil but not in Hemp *Seed* Oil. The CBD Oil that is generally consumed, however, is an entirely separate extract all on its own.

CBD Oil that is extracted to be used as a health supplement is extracted in a manner that allows it to stay pure and free of THC and other radicals that may take away from the quality of the oil itself.

12th *thing you need know...*

The way CBD Oil is extracted from the plant is crucial in ensuring the quality of the oil is kept in tact. When not extracted efficiently, CBD Oil will be inferior, and therefore will not have as great of an impact on supporting individuals in experiencing the health benefits. The correct way to extract CBD Oil is by the way of carbon dioxide (CO_2) to maintain its integrity.

What is A Cannabinoid?

13th *thing you need know...*

A Cannabinoid is known to be the primary chemical compound that was discovered in the Hemp and Cannabis plants.

14th *thing you need know...*

Cannabinoids were discovered in the 1940s with scientists originally discovering CBD and CBN in the trichomes of the Hemp plant. THC was not discovered until much later in 1964. Scientists have continued to research the plant for the past seventy plus years, finding approximately 111 more cannabinoids since.

Chapter 2: Why Should I Use CBD Oil?

This chapter is going to tell you all of the reasons why you would want to use CBD Oil. This oil was derived for the benefit of its medicinal values, so everything you learn in this chapter will highlight these benefits, and support you in understanding how valuable this oil truly is.

Why is CBD Oil Good For You?

15th thing you need know...

Unlike other medicines that are commonly prescribed for the same uses, CBD Oil has nothing in it that will make you feel "high".

Many conventional medicines prescribed for the same purpose that CBD Oil can be used for, often produce a high feeling, or otherwise, alter the personality and state of the individual in a way that may make them feel like they are distant from themselves.

CBD Oil, however, will not create any of these effects. It works within your body without having any psychoactive impact on you.

16th thing you need know...

CBD Oil is considered to be good for you because it is a whole plant medicine. Whole plant medicines have continued to grow in popularity over the years, assisting individuals in choosing safer alternatives to conventional medicines.

Additionally, because they are whole plants without any additives, they are believed to be easier and safer for the body to digest and use without producing negative side effects.

17th thing you need know...

Many conventional medicines prescribed for the same reasons as CBD Oil are known to have a long list of unhealthy side effects. Many of these often include the side effect of "death."

CBD Oil contains very few side effects. However, the side effects which can occur through using CBD Oil will be discussed in *"Chapter 5: Side effects of CBD Oil."*

18th thing you need know...

CBD Oil is known to promote emotional homeostasis. This is a state whereby users minimize the ups and downs that are often incurred by emotional upsets, which are known to be common in many ailments, including anything from as simple as chronic pain to as drastic as a terminal illness.

Taking a supplement that can support your well-being while also promote your emotional homeostasis means that you will experience less stress. When you experience less stress, not only do you feel better emotionally, but your body also has a stronger chance to fight against anything that may be ailing it. Stress in itself can be an illness. So, no longer having to face these stressors can have a major positive impact on your overall health.

19th thing you need know...

If you are interested in the environment and want to support your own health in the process, CBD Oil is a great choice.

CBD Oil is a highly sustainable product, which as mentioned previously is derived from a plant that has many uses. That means that the same plant that was grown to produce your medicine is also being used to create fibers to be used in sustainable and ethical cloth and paper products. This also means that fewer crops have to be grown and the crops are less damaging to the environment.

20th thing you need know...

Hemp plants are ready to be harvested much quicker than other medicines. It is easier to produce higher amounts of Hemp plants from smaller crop fields.

21st thing you need know...

CBD Oil is known to be an antioxidant, meaning that it can support your body in eliminating free radicals.

Free radicals in the body have been known to promote the onset of many diseases and ailments, such as cancer. Eliminating them is great for supporting your overall long-term health and preventing these diseases from having the capacity to develop in your system.

22nd thing you need know...

Because of its nature, CBD Oil has the capacity to treat many things. This means that while you may be taking it for one specific reason, it will also be working on other symptoms within your body. So, while you experience relief from your primary concern, you will also experience greater health in other areas as a result of this medicine.

It is one of the few medicines you can take that will have many positive benefits, as opposed to strictly treating the specific condition you are focused on.

23rd thing you need know...

Unlike many conventional medicines, CBD Oil can be taken in many different ways. As a result, you can easily get it into your system in whatever way works best for you. This versatility makes it excellent for treating many ailments because you can get it directly to the source of the symptom quickly and in the most effective way possible in a way that is also more comfortable for you.

24th thing you need know...

Instead of reaching for over-the-counter medicines like ibuprofen and acetaminophen, many clinicians believe that the future includes CBD Oil being used as a standard-practice supplement in everyone's cupboards. The aforementioned medicines, when ingested too frequently, have been shown to deteriorate the stomach lining and increase problematic symptoms such as heartburn and acid reflux.

Using CBD Oil as an alternative would likely prove to be safer and more effective for those who need relief from symptoms such as headaches or general muscle aches and pains.

25th thing you need know...

CBD Oil has been known to counteract the impacts of THC. This is why many recreational marijuana growers will minimize CBD content while maximizing THC content. It allows people to experience greater psychoactive effects. This is also why having 0.3% or less THC in your CBD Oil is not a bad thing. The CBD will counteract it and prevent you from experiencing psychoactive effects.

Is it Safe?

26th thing you need know...

Although CBD Oil is praised for being highly natural, some individuals may not be able to take it due to it poorly interacting with other medicines that they may already be taking.

There may be other health-related issues that reduce the safeness of CBD Oil, so it is always a good idea to talk to your healthcare practitioner before ingesting any prescribed supplement.

If you are with a practitioner who tends to have conservative views, they may immediately rule out CBD Oil simply because they do not believe in using it at all. If this is the case, you may benefit from going to a doctor who is CBD-informed and able to genuinely support you in making a choice that is right for you, versus making a choice that is based on your healthcare practitioner's morals.

27th thing you need know...

CBD Oil is a natural plant extract. In its purest form it can be unsafe for your body. This is why those who sell CBD Oil will dilute it with carrier oils such as fractionated coconut oil or jojoba oil. It can then be safely applied or ingested without producing negative or harmful side effects to you. When buying CBD Oil, ensure that you thoroughly research how the oil has been extracted and what carrier oils have been used, as this can also affect the quality of the oil.

It is important that you never apply pure CBD Oil to your body or ingest it, as it may cause severe damage. All natural plant extracts, including standard essential oils such as peppermint oil or eucalyptus oil, are extremely strong and can cause irritation, burns, or other damage to any part of the body that it may come into contact with.

28th thing you need know...

Some medicines are known to have side effects that can actually enhance the symptom that the user is attempting to avoid. For example, some anti-depressants are known to increase symptoms of depression and the tendency of experiencing suicidal thoughts, thus putting the user at a greater risk of suicide.

CBD Oil, on the other hand, does not have any side effects like this. Typically, the worst side effect is that it will not work or that you need your dosage adjusted.

Therefore, using CBD Oil may be safer because it reduces the risk of facing challenging side effects that may be detrimental or fatal to the user.

29th thing you need know...

Although it cannot combine with all medicines, most medicines are not impacted by the use of CBD Oil. This means, you can use CBD Oil as a safe alternative to pain medications to help you alleviate symptoms that you may experience from other medical treatments.

This has been especially popular amongst cancer patients who may be experiencing negative symptoms and side effects from harsh cancer treatments such as radiation. Taking CBD Oil can minimize these symptoms while allowing the radiation to successfully complete what it was put in the body to do.

30th thing you need know...

CBD Oil is believed to have neuroprotective properties, meaning that it can support and protect the neurological system. To those who are struggling with neurological conditions such as seizures or multiple sclerosis, CBD Oil can provide great relief from the symptoms of these conditions.

31st thing you need know...

31st thing you need know...

CBD Oil is believed to have a positive impact on the circulatory system. When taken in the correct dosage, it can lower high blood pressure and promote a healthier functioning heart. It is likely that the stress- and anxiety-reducing properties of the oil are responsible for lowering blood pressure.

Common Uses

32nd thing you need know...

CBD Oil is known to fight against cancer. CBD and other cannabinoids found in the Cannabis plant have been proven to have an anti-tumor effect, and are also known to support the fight with standard treatments.

In a recent study, CBD was successful in stopping multiple different cervical cancer cells in a patient. It has also increased tumor cell death in both colon cancer and leukemia. It is also known to be promising in combination therapies that many medics use for breast and prostate cancers.

Combination therapy means that it can be used alongside other conventional or alternative therapies, working together to promote the reversal of tumors and cancer cells in patients who have been diagnosed with varying types of cancer.

33rd thing you need know...

Many people use CBD Oil due to the fact that this oil is incredible for relieving pain. This analgesic (a supplement with pain-relieving effects) interacts with receptors in your brain and immune system to support your body in alleviating pain and reducing any inflammation that may be contributing to the pain. Due to the nature of this supplement, these benefits are often experienced with zero side effects.

34th thing you need know...

One of the most incredible and notable features of CBD Oil is its ability to minimize and eliminate seizures from patients who were previously experiencing many.

Some producers and distributors of CBD Oil

have noted that they have witnessed patients, who experienced more than 100 seizures a day, have absolutely none for several weeks on end after using CBD Oil.

The oil has even been noted to stop a seizure from happening within minutes of symptoms beginning.

35th thing you need know...

Anxiety is something that a large portion of the population faces. The Anxiety and Depression Association of America (ADAA) estimates that more than 40 million Americans who are over the age of 18 are impacted or affected by anxiety. This accounts for approximately 18% of the entire American population.

CBD Oil has shown promising effects in minimizing and eliminating anxiety disorder, even for those experiencing crippling anxiety that prevents them from leading a typical lifestyle with basic activities.

CBD Oil works on anxiety by relaxing an individual in their limbic and paralimbic brain areas. Again, CBD Oil can stunt the effects of a panic or anxiety attack within minutes of an individual consuming the oil.

36th thing you need know...

A lesser-known benefit of CBD Oil is that it is capable of supporting individuals in reducing their risk of developing diabetes.

Recently, Neuropharmacology released a study that showed that CBD Oil prevented 67% of non-obese diabetes-prone female mice from developing the disease, whereas, 100% of untreated mice with the same likelihood of developing the disease did go on to develop the disease.

There are still studies being done to show how effective this is for adult humans, though the results are looking very promising.

37th thing you need know...

Many individuals in modern society face a wide range of sleep-related issues. From experiencing restless sleep that results in them waking feeling un-rested to full-blown insomnia.

One of the "side effects" of CBD Oil is promoting a better rest in adults, sometimes leading them to feel sleepy after taking the supplement. This means that instead of using addictive and potentially damaging medicines that can cause false positive sleep patterns, you can use a safe alternative through this holistic supplement. CBD Oil has been found to promote a healthier and sounder sleep pattern without creating any addictions or harming you in any way.

38th thing you need know...

One interesting benefit many users claim to gain from CBD Oil is that this supplement reduces acne.

Acne is believed to develop in individuals for many reasons, ranging from genetics to bacteria or even underlying conditions.

Science has recently shown that using CBD Oil through topical application has the potential to improve acne conditions, likely as a result of its anti-inflammatory effects. So, using CBD Oil can help reduce and reverse problematic anxiety in individuals who may be struggling to keep their face clear and free of acne.

39th thing you need know...

CBD Oil has shown to have antipsychotic properties. While it is not yet being issued in standard practice, many studies have shown that CBD Oil has the capacity to minimize psychotic episodes, such as those linked to schizophrenia or other mental disorders that produce psychotic symptoms.

Using this supplement has shown promising benefits in reducing psychotic symptoms and episodes, supporting those who have been diagnosed with these types of mental disorders in their ability to lead a higher quality life, free of challenging and problematic symptoms that can prevent them from living a typical life.

40th thing you need know...

Many addictions therapists have been using CBD Oil as a way to help individuals who are quitting hard drugs such as heroin and methamphetamine to reduce difficult symptoms of withdrawal.

In studies that have been done to investigate the successful benefits of this medicine, researchers have shown that CBD Oil can support drug-addicted individuals in reducing difficult symptoms as well as in preventing dependency and drug-seeking behaviors. In other words, those who were using CBD Oil as a part of their treatment were able to go several days, or longer, without actively seeking out drugs to support their addiction.

41st thing you need know...

Quitting smoking is another great benefit of using CBD Oil. Much like with supporting individuals in quitting their addictions to harder drugs, CBD Oil can also support individuals in quitting their addiction to cigarettes.

Research studies showed that those who used placebo inhalers experienced no change in their overall cigarette consumption, whereas, those who used CBD Oil smoked nearly 40% fewer cigarettes on average each day.

42nd thing you need know...

Fibromyalgia is a chronic pain condition that has no known cause and few tried and true remedies that work for everyone who takes them. It is a fairly mysterious condition that cannot be treated by others.

CBD Oil has been shown to be a powerful pain

remedy and symptom remedy for those diagnosed with fibromyalgia. In studies that have been done, virtually everyone who was put on the CBD Oil treatment saw significantly reduced symptoms, with some of them even going on to live symptom-free.

43rd *thing you need know...*

Post Traumatic Stress Disorder (PTSD) is a highly complex form of advanced anxiety that is experienced by those who have been in traumatic situations. Many think of post-war veterans when they think of PTSD, but the reality is that this disorder actually impacts far more than just them.

Those who have been exposed to varying degrees of abuse throughout their life have also been shown to develop PTSD as a result as well. In these individuals, using CBD Oil has shown to have a profound impact on supporting them in living symptom-free.

Those who take it have been shown to experience great relief, thus making it a great potential treatment for those living with PTSD. Due to the anti-anxiety, anti-stress, anti-inflammatory, and antipsychotic effects of CBD Oil, it supports

those living with PTSD in experiencing a more
mentally stable environment for them.

44th thing you need know...

Research and studies have also been done with
those who have been living with either Crohn's
disease or irritable bowel syndrome (IBS).

Scientists have discovered that CBD Oil may
have a powerful impact on supporting the relief
of symptoms related to these two conditions.

Due to its anti-inflammatory properties and the
way CBD Oil interacts with the part of your body
responsible for controlling gut function, CBD Oil
has been shown to support individuals with
either of these conditions in being able to pass
bowel movements with greater ease and less
symptomatic pain and/or suffering.

45th thing you need know...

Multiple Sclerosis is a disease that is chronic and
progressive. It damages nerves in your brain and
spinal cord, leading to the loss of use of many
muscles and body parts. Those with this disease
are known to have difficulty speaking and using
muscular coordination. They also struggle with

blurred vision and severe fatigue as a result of the disease.

Studies have shown that using CBD Oil can greatly improve symptoms relating to this disease, potentially even reversing the symptoms and protecting the body against multiple sclerosis altogether. Using CBD Oil may help those with multiple sclerosis regain control over their muscles and live a better life following treatment than they would have without the use of CBD Oil.

46th *thing you need know...*

Rheumatoid arthritis is a painful form of arthritis that damages bones and joints and can lead to a malformed body over time.

Due to CBD Oil having anti-inflammatory effects and inflammation is one of the leading symptoms and causes of degeneration with rheumatoid arthritis, taking this oil may support those living with this condition to experience reduced symptoms.

It has been shown to decrease joint destruction and slow down disease progression, allowing those with a diagnosis of rheumatoid arthritis to lead a longer, happier, and healthier life.

47th *thing you need know...*

Although the research into this one is not as extensive, studies have shown that individuals who are suffering from broken bones have healed faster with the use of CBD Oil than without.

Bone growth is considered to be one of the benefits of this supplement. Studies are continuing to be done to see if this supplement can support individuals in having improved bone health overall, potentially contributing to faster broken bones healing as well as fewer symptomatic side effects of osteoporosis.

48th *thing you need know...*

Psoriasis is a painful and uncomfortable skin condition that results in the extremely dry flaky skin on those who suffer with it.

When used topically in an ointment, cream, serum, or lotion, CBD Oil has been shown to support individuals in minimizing their symptoms of psoriasis and experiencing greater skin health. Since this condition can be itchy, painful, and embarrassing, it is extremely helpful to those suffering to experience freedom from their problematic symptoms.

49th thing you need know...

Dyskinesia and Restless Leg Syndrome (RLS) are two conditions that cause an involuntary muscle movement in those who are struggling with the conditions.

CBD, when combined with a TRPV-1 blocker, has been shown to reduce symptoms of these conditions, supporting individuals in minimizing involuntary muscle movement and thus having greater control over their muscles in general.

50th thing you need know...

Due to our poor diets and the way we live our lives; many of us live with some form of a gastrointestinal disease that can cause nausea and vomiting, as well as decreased appetite.

CBD Oil has been shown to relieve these symptoms and support individuals struggling with poor gut health in experiencing an increased appetite so they can nourish their bodies with ease.

As a side note, THC has also been a proven effective method in supporting the same benefits. In fact, some clinics will prescribe "dronabinol", which is a medicine made with THC, to those who are suffering. However, clinics are showing that CBD has greater promise in supporting good health over THC as it contains fewer side effects which can affect the patient.

51st thing you need know...

In people who have injuries to their spinal cord, CBD Oil is great in helping to treat both the nerve damage and the symptomatic pain experienced by this injury.

For those who have suffered from traumatic accidents, this may be revolutionary in providing non-addictive pain relief to victims.

52nd thing you need know...

CBD Oil is in the process of being studied to understand how it may help individuals who have experienced a stroke.

The oil has shown to be effective in studies where

symptoms of a stroke, such as nerve damage, is being treated and reversed with the use of CBD Oil.

While this is still in the very early stages of research, the findings have been promising in showing that individuals are regaining painless use of their limbs and muscles with CBD Oil treatment following a stroke.

Chapter 3: How Do I Take CBD Oil?

Taking CBD Oil clearly has many benefits and positive outcomes for those who use it. However, you may still be wondering *how* to use it. One incredible thing about this supplement is that it is extremely versatile in how you can take it and how much you can take of it. Typically, the way CBD Oil is used depends on what type of ailment you are treating. Here are some facts that you should know about on how you can use CBD Oil.

Topically

53rd *thing you need know...*

Because it is a natural plant extract, pure CBD Oil should never be taken topically without first being diluted into some form of tincture, lotion, balm, or otherwise. Pure CBD Oil applied directly to the skin may cause irritation, taking away from the healing benefits that it is otherwise known for having.

54th *thing you need know...*

Most distributors of CBD Oil will have a variety of different topical CBD Oil products that you can use. These products are made differently so that they target different purposes as well as with varying dosages.

It is always a good idea to seek support in discovering which one will work best for your needs unless you are already educated on what exactly you are looking for.

55th thing you need know...

Topical CBD Oil products do not have the same affect that the ingestible CBD Oil products do. This means that they are faster working and that you get a more focused healing benefit for your desired symptom. For example, if you have psoriasis, applying CBD Oil topically will work directly on psoriasis, whereas, ingesting it would work on your entire body and take significantly longer to improve your psoriasis.

56th thing you need know...

Applying CBD Oil topically is the least invasive method for using CBD Oil.

Both ingesting it and inhaling it will work

directly on your entire body, whereas applying it topically focuses primarily on the issue it has been applied to.

Furthermore, because CBD Oil in topical products interacts with the CB2 receptors near your skin, they activate the endocannabinoid system. This means that unlike other varieties of topical treatments, CBD Oil will never actually enter your bloodstream through topical products.

57th thing you need know...

Most topical products will advise you to "apply liberally" because human skin is known to have a low absorption rate for cannabinoids. While this works great to prevent it from entering the bloodstream, it also means that you need to use a lot in order for the skin to actually absorb enough of the product for it to be beneficial.

58th thing you need know...

Topical CBD products are not just used on skin-related issues. They are also used on joint-related issues and acute pain, such as with rheumatoid arthritis or fibromyalgia. Applying it directly to the pain itself can cause quicker relief, making it more effective for some of these symptoms than actually ingesting the CBD Oil.

59th *thing you need know...*

Some chronic conditions, such as fibromyalgia, will use CBD Oil through ingestible products to maintain ongoing symptom relief as well as use topical treatments to work directly on symptoms that may flare up despite the ongoing use of CBD Oil supplements.

This supports individuals in experiencing nearly total symptom relief. This combination treatment may be used on a variety of conditions that cause pain or other acute physical symptoms.

Ingested

60th *thing you need know...*

Ingesting CBD Oil tends to be one of the easiest ways for beginners or children to take CBD oil for their symptoms. This is the most commonly prescribed method for those who are using CBD Oil to treat a condition.

When you swallow a CBD oil pill, you are swallowing concentrated oil that is then passed through the digestive system and metabolized by the liver. This allows it to enter into your bloodstream where it begins to work on your symptoms. This is the same way most daily vitamins are delivered into your system.

61st thing you need know...

Because the process of ingesting oil requires the capsule to first be passed through the digestive system, ingesting oil can take up to two hours before full effects are experienced. However, many people report experiencing positive effects from it within minutes of taking the capsule.

This means that ingesting CBD Oil through a concentrated capsule form can have slow-release type effects on users, allowing them to experience symptom relief for up to four hours after taking a single dosage.

62nd thing you need know...

If you prefer not to swallow a capsule, CBD Oil can also come in a small pill that you place under your tongue and melt with your saliva. This allows the oil to enter directly into your bloodstream, giving you quicker symptom relief lasting for several hours.

For people with random and quick onset of symptoms, this can be a great way for quickly alleviating those symptoms without having to wait for the digestive system to break down the capsule and digest the oil.

63rd *thing you need know...*

Another way that many people ingest CBD Oil is through eating what dispensaries often call "gourmet treats."

These are baked goods which are made with CBD Oil to deliver the same results through digestion but in a way that eliminates the swallowing of a capsule or the need to melt a pill under your tongue.

For some people, eating smaller rations of food made with CBD Oil throughout the day can allow the oil to continually deliver consistent results all day long. Some foods that are regularly made with CBD Oil include varieties of yogurt, popcorn, and cooking oil that can be mixed into salad dressing recipes or used as finishing oil for various dishes, butter, coffee, smoothies or pasta sauce.

There are many varieties of edibles these days. You can find anything that works best for you and consume that to receive the great benefits of CBD Oil without having to take it in pill form.

64th thing you need know...

If you are taking CBD Oil in capsule form, the dosage can easily be adjusted by the dispensary. This means that you can request lower dosage and higher dosage CBD Oil capsules that allow you to receive your best results from the supplement without feeling like you are overdoing it.

These can be considered akin to "regular strength" and "extra strength" supplements for those who are using them this way.

65th thing you need know...

Other forms of CBD Oil that are not edibles but are not capsules either include tinctures and concentrates. These are unique creations with CBD Oil that are taken orally and allow the CBD Oil to almost immediately enter the endocannabinoid system in the body so that you begin to experience immediate effects.

Tinctures are great because they can be flavored, making it more enjoyable to take. Concentrates can be used for higher dosages and quick-relief from symptoms.

Vaporized

66th thing you need know...

CBD oil can be vaporized, which is one of the leading reasons why many people may confuse it for THC or Marijuana and fall under the false belief that it can make you "high."

As you already know from Chapter 1, there are key differences between CBD Oil and Marijuana or THC Oil. Vaporizing CBD Oil will not deliver any form of high unless the oil has THC in it. When you vaporize CBD Oil, you are still taking the same thing. You are simply delivering it to your system by a different means.

67th thing you need know...

Vaporizing CBD Oil was one of the first methods for taking CBD Oil before it was researched in depth and new ways were discovered.

Researchers later looked at the plant and searched for new ways that they could isolate the CBD Oil compound and create other methods for taking the supplement that did not involve vaporizing.

68th thing you need know...

Many people prefer to vaporize CBD Oil because it enters the lungs and then immediately enters the bloodstream along with your oxygen. This results in quick relief from symptoms which may not experience relief from topical treatments and may take too long to relieve through ingesting it.

69th thing you need know...

Vaporizing is not the same as smoking. When you vaporize something, enough heat is being applied to it that it essentially becomes a steam. The CBD compound is then transported into your body through this steam.

When you smoke something, you burn it to the point that it is smoking and it enters your body through the smoke. While smoke has been shown to have carcinogenic effects, vapor has not. This means that vaporizing CBD Oil refrains from burning off some of it and wasting it, as well as prevents you from experiencing adverse side effects of the smoke.

People who have chronic asthma or lung conditions will often vaporize CBD Oil for instant relief and no adverse side effects that may come from smoking.

70th thing you need know...

Vaporizing CBD Oil requires you to use a pure form of CBD Oil concentrate. This is the kind that you may ingest, but that you typically do not want to apply directly to your skin.

You want to make sure you are using pure CBD Oil because you do not want to be vaporizing and inhaling any other ingredients that may be harmful to your health.

If you plan on vaporizing, make sure your dispensary knows this, so that they can administer the proper form of oil to you, so that you do not experience any harmful or adverse reactions.

71st thing you need know...

Vaporizers come in many shapes and sizes. You can purchase pen-style vaporizers that are small and easy to transport, portable vaporizers that are larger but still easy to transport, and desktop or stationary vaporizers that are much larger and tend to deliver higher dosages with a plug-in feature that will vaporize the oil for you.

These vaporizers may deliver you the vapor via a tube, a bag or a balloon, or as a direct draw vaporizer. They tend to be heated with conduction, convection, or infrared heating systems that are designed to control the output temperature so as to heat your oil just enough to be vaporized but not so much to be burnt and turned into a smoke.

72nd *thing you need know...*

Some vaporizers are made in a way that allows them to vaporize dry herbs. This means that your dispensary may distribute a piece of the cannabis plant that is high in CBD content but features little to no THC content.

Remember, in order for these supplements to be legal, they must have less than 0.3% THC in them. This means that if your distributor gives you something like this, you are still not going to get high from the herb.

However, it is still important to communicate with your distributor as some do carry herbs that are high in THC as well for other medicinal values.

73rd *thing you need know...*

Despite other delivery systems becoming available, many believe that vaporizing should still be the most commonly used form for delivering CBD Oil to a patient's system. This is because topical creams require a high amount of product in order to be effective, and ingested CBD Oil can take longer to activate.

Furthermore, using a vaporizer is much safer than smoking the herb, thus making it the safest and most effective method for delivering the CBD into your body.

Chapter 4: Who Should Take CBD Oil?

In this chapter, we are going to discover facts about who can safely take CBD Oil and who cannot. Naturally, you want to make sure that you are safe to take it to refrain from experiencing any negative side effects. This is simply common knowledge when planning on taking any new supplements or medicinal products!

General Facts

74th thing you need know...

Based on research, the majority of individuals can take CBD Oil and not face risks of having any major side effects as a result of taking the supplement.

This is one of the safest and most versatile supplements on the market that can support a variety of medicinal causes without causing adverse side effects to various age groups.

75th thing you need know...

In addition to humans being able to take CBD Oil, veterinarians and researchers have begun to realize that CBD Oil can also be used by animals for many causes.

In particular, dogs with epilepsy or senior dogs with arthritis have been shown to have great positive reactions to the supplement. It has also been tested for a number of other ailments in animals and has shown to have the same positive effect.

It is important to note, however, that using other forms of cannabis including marijuana is not safe for animals so refrain from using anything without the support or assistance of your vet.

Also, how animals take the oil should be monitored to refrain from giving it to them in a way that may be harmful. In this case, the method of delivery would be harmful and not the supplement itself.

Children

76th thing you need know...

Because THC and CBD are not the same, many

children can safely take CBD supplements without experiencing any adverse reactions.

Frequently, CBD Oil is used to treat conditions such as chronic pain conditions and epilepsy in children.

77th *thing you need know...*

Not all CBD Oil is made the same. For this reason, you need to ensure that you are getting your CBD over-the-counter from a trusted dispensary.

CBD Oil that you purchase online may have some degree of THC in it which is not recommended or advised for consumption by children. While CBD will not create any psychoactive symptoms, THC will if it is present in larger amounts and this can be dangerous for children.

Although the FDA does work hard to eliminate any untrustworthy online dealers who may be selling CBD Oil with higher-than-allowed levels of THC in it, it does not mean that every seller will be properly screened and shut down if necessary.

It is advised that you take all necessary precautions, especially with children, to refrain them from having any adverse reactions.

78th thing you need know...

Especially with children, consulting with a trained healthcare professional is important.

While CBD Oil itself is relatively safe and has no instances of death or serious lasting side effects, giving it to young children may not always be safe.

Some doctors may advise against it and instead offer other therapies. That being said, always take the time to make sure you understand your doctor's overall stance on CBD Oil.

Many conservative doctors are still morally against it and therefore will suggest that absolutely no one should be using this supplement. Working together with a CBD-informed healthcare professional can support you in making the right choice.

79th thing you need know...

Children who live with Autism, Sensory

Processing Disorder (SPD,) ADD or ADHD or other disorders that are especially challenging in youth, having a CBD supplement can help manage symptoms and support the child in feeling more capable of "fitting in" to their environment.

CBD Oil has been shown to minimize the stress that the child may face and support them in feeling a sense of belonging in their environment.

80th thing you need know...

Currently, CBD Oil is not legal in every state. For that reason, you need to be careful to look over state laws and only purchase when it is legal for your state.

Taking the oil as a consenting adult in a state where it is illegal can be incriminating, never mind giving the supplement to a youth.

Make sure that you know the laws and that you follow them accordingly to refrain from being incriminated for using this supplement.

Adults

81st thing you need know...

CBD Oil is not necessarily the cheapest medication available, though you can find places that will make it more affordable.

Most healthcare insurance will not cover the purchase, so you will need to purchase CBD Oil out of your own pocket. That being said, there are some programs that certain dispensaries are enrolled in where you can enroll to make the supplement cheaper for you to purchase.

82nd thing you need know...

Just like with children, adults who are considering using CBD Oil need to consult a healthcare practitioner.

While CBD Oil in itself is not dangerous, having a trained professional supporting you in finding the right way to deliver it into your system and how much to take is important.

Someone who knows what they are doing will support you in using enough that you can feel the positive effects without overdoing it and wasting your money or risking your health.

Seniors

83rd *thing you need know...*

In seniors who are facing common symptoms of aging, such as arthritis and other pain-related symptoms, using CBD Oil is considered to be a safer alternative to having other medicines available for these conditions.

CBD Oil can provide the same degree of symptom relief without other adverse reactions that may, in some cases, be even harsher to seniors.

84th *thing you need know...*

Seniors tend to be more at risk for developing diseases such as Alzheimer's and Parkinson's disease. Due to the nature of CBD Oil being anti-inflammatory, having neuroprotective properties, and being able to calm and regulate muscle function to prevent involuntary movement, CBD Oil has proven effective in helping to relieve symptoms related to these conditions.

In the past, these conditions have caused severe

discomfort and inconveniences to the individuals suffering from them, so having effective relief that could restore their quality of life is important.

85th thing you need know...

Later in life, many seniors find themselves being faced with a medicine cabinet that is filled with a variety of different medications. Each one of those medications often comes with their own long-list of potential side effects.

Since the older bodies of seniors are more vulnerable, they are at higher risk of facing these side effects. Many seniors even have medicines specifically prescribed to treat the symptoms of other side effects. Furthermore, not all of these medicines are covered by insurances, resulting in seniors likely having to pay enormous amounts for their medicine.

While CBD Oil is not necessarily a cheaper alternative, it may come in at around the same amount per month. Also, it is one single supplement as opposed to having many. Seniors would not have to treat for symptoms of other medicines and instead could enjoy a higher quality of life simply through the use of one single supplement, as opposed to a medicine cabinet full of them.

86th *thing you need know...*

Although CBD Oil cannot prevent death, it can make the process of dealing with terminal illnesses a lot more bearable for those going through them.

For seniors who are regularly developing terminal illnesses having access to CBD Oil as a part of their therapy may make their elder years more enjoyable by reducing problematic symptoms and giving them the opportunity to enjoy those later years.

87th *thing you need know...*

Another fear that some have in later years that is not necessarily a symptom of taking medicine but more so a symptom of aging is accidentally taking a double-dosage of medicine.

Taking a supplement that has the potential to provide the same relief but is not *as dangerous* if it is taken in a double-dosage can provide a great peace of mind to seniors.

Since CBD Oil cannot produce overdoses, seniors are not at risk for accidentally taking a potentially fatal dose of medicine. Still, seniors should consult with a healthcare practitioner before using CBD Oil just to be on the side of caution.

Chapter 5: Side Effects of CBD Oil

Despite being touted for not having any problematic side effects *for most people,* CBD Oil has been reported to cause some mild, non-life threatening side effects in those who take it.

Occasionally, depending on the medical condition of those taking it, it may not be considered a safe supplement. Here are some facts that you should know about the side effects of CBD Oil.

Medicinal Considerations

88th thing you need know...

Those who have problems with lower blood pressure should not take CBD Oil as it can further lower blood pressure and may put them at risk of cardiac arrest.

If you have chronically low blood pressure or find yourself struggling with heart health in this way, taking CBD Oil may not be the best choice for you.

89th thing you need know...

If you are taking drugs such as steroids, calcium channel blockers, HIV antivirals, antibiotics, beta blockers, NSAIDs, oral hypoglycemic agents, or other medicines, taking CBD Oil can react with these medicines and cause negative symptoms.

It is important that if you are taking any other medicines, even temporarily, that you are transparent with your doctor about using CBD Oil and that you refrain from using the oil in combination with any medicines which may be deemed unsafe to use with CBD Oil.

90th thing you need know...

The way people metabolize CBD is vastly different, this means that people who are taking CBD Oil need to be monitored early on for symptoms to make sure that their dosage is correct.

When the dosage is correct, there should be no problematic symptoms from the CBD Oil *and* all or most of your symptoms should be minimized or alleviated.

91st *thing you need know...*

While some medicines work adversely with CBD Oil, some actually work well together with it. This is called combination therapy.

In order to discover whether or not CBD Oil will work well with the medications you are currently using, you should chat with a CBD-informed doctor who can support you in making an informed choice.

Symptomatic Side Effects

92nd *thing you need know...*

Despite CBD Oil being known to treat anxiety and depression, some individuals may experience increased anxiety and depression after using CBD.

While the cause for this is not entirely known, it is believed to be in relation to the fact that CBD Oil slows things down, such as your circulatory system, which may trigger symptoms of depression or anxiety in some users.

93rd thing you need know...

Proper CBD Oil should not have enough THC in it to react within your body. However, some individuals have shown to experience psychosis after using CBD Oil.

This may be caused by being sensitive toward the compound, or it may be because they purchased it from an untrustworthy source and it had higher than legal levels of THC in it.

It is important to make sure that you are monitored by a trained healthcare professional when using this supplement and that you are purchasing it from safe and trusted sources.

94th thing you need know...

Some individuals who take CBD Oil may find themselves experiencing nausea. In most cases, this comes from taking a higher-than-needed dosage.

For others, the concentration of the oil may be too much for their body. Switching to an alternative delivery method or choosing a different supplement or medicine altogether may be necessary for these individuals.

95th thing you need know...

In severe cases, CBD Oil may cause vomiting in individuals. Vomiting is generally caused by the body struggling to digest it or by the CBD Oil irritating the lining of the stomach.

If this is happening, avoid taking it again until you can communicate with your healthcare practitioner. It may be because you have too high of a dosage, or it may be because you are sensitive to the oil and need to choose an alternative method for relieving symptoms.

96th thing you need know...

CBD Oil is known to be great for supporting individuals in having better sleep, hence, why many use it to ward off symptoms of restless sleep or insomnia. That being said, drowsiness is known to be one of the side effects of CBD Oil.

If you are not taking it for the purpose of sleeping better at night and you feel that the drowsiness is becoming problematic, you may be able to switch your dosage or take it differently to avoid this side effect.

97th thing you need know...

Some individuals who take CBD Oil report having a dry mouth after taking it. Ingesting enough water to keep yourself healthily hydrated and sucking on cough drops or small hard candies can help keep saliva in your mouth and prevent dry mouth.

 Otherwise, if it is extremely problematic, you might consider switching your dosage to avoid this symptom altogether.

98th thing you need know...

Some people who take CBD Oil find that they get dizzy after taking it. This may be due to having a lower blood pressure after taking the medicine.

If you experience dizziness, be sure to move slowly between lying down, sitting, and standing positions to avoid falling over. Refrain from taking any further medicine until you have communicated with your doctor. If this is a symptom of abnormally low blood pressure, continuing to take the medicine could result in harmful effects.

99th thing you need know...

The exact reasoning is unknown, but some individuals who use CBD Oil find themselves experiencing diarrhea afterward. This may be due to the digestive system struggling to break it down or relaxing too much.

If this happens, be sure to drink more fluids. If it persists, communicate this with your doctor and see if your dosage can be adjusted to avoid this side effect.

100th thing you need know...

Generally, people who take CBD Oil find themselves feeling an increased appetite.

Alternatively, if you are experiencing early symptoms of nausea, you may feel a decreased appetite. If you feel that your appetite has changed too much for you to maintain a healthy level of intake or like you are consistently eating too much, consider talking to your doctor to have your dosage adjusted.

101st thing you need know...

Some individuals who have Parkinson's disease have noticed increased tremors as opposed to decreased tremors when taking CBD Oil. For that reason, it may not be effective for all cases of Parkinson's disease. Still, some individuals experience great relief as a result of it.

Conclusion

Congratulations on reading *"CBD: 101 Things You Need to Know About CBD Oil"*!

This fun yet comprehensive guide was designed to provide you with 101 things to inform you about CBD Oil and why it is all the rage in modern culture. Everyone is talking about it, the government is legalizing it, and many are experiencing life-changing results from it. It is a seriously powerful supplement that has the power to change the way we face our health in a really positive way.

I hope that in reading this guide, you were able to get a better understanding of what CBD Oil is, where it comes from, and why it is used. I hope you were also able to learn about the pros and cons, and much more information to support you in understanding this supplement in greater detail.

Whether you are brand new to the supplement or you have been reading about it for some time, I set the intention of making this guide a one-stop source for you to learn as much as possible in one simple location.

The next step is for you to consider how CBD Oil may benefit you or the loved ones. If you find that you are leaning towards taking the supplement, communicate with a certified healthcare practitioner who is CBD-informed and who can support you in making the right choice. Always be sure to be transparent with your current health conditions and any medications you are taking as you never want to have accidental adverse reactions due to withholding the truth from your doctor.

Furthermore, make sure that you pay attention to getting your oil from a safe and trusted dispensary who knows what they are doing. Take the time to ask them how their oils are made, where they come from, and what they do to verify that they are as safe as they say they are.

You want to make sure that anything going into your body is safe for you. If they are a safe and trustworthy dispensary, they will be willing to answer any questions you have and should be happy to support you in feeling confident in your choice.

Lastly, if you enjoyed this book, I ask that you please take the time to review it on Amazon. Your honest feedback would be greatly appreciated.

Thank you.

Made in the USA
San Bernardino, CA
07 April 2020

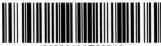
66833102R00042